HOW TO LOSE 21 POUNDS OF BODY FAT IN A MONTH EXPOSED!

BY: SHAWN BIGGS

8 Keto Diet Myths and Facts What You Need to Know

Keeping your body in ketosis is the main purpose of the keto diet. This diet plan includes healthy vegetables and fats, low carbs, and adequate protein. This diet plan specifically advises against the intake of sugary and high carbs foods. There are different types of the keto diet and they are high-protein diet, targeted, cyclical, standard ketogenic. The stages of the keto diet usually depend on the intake of carbohydrates. The standard ketogenic diet is a diet high in protein, high in fat, and low in carbs.

If you want to lose excess body weight very fast, you can come in the middle of a ketogenic diet which will be fruitful. The keto diet is more popular for rapid weight loss which promises to reduce excess weight in a short period. However, according to most people, diet is not a magical way through which you can suddenly notice physical changes. Like other diet plans, it is a matter of time which is done through some rules and sacrifices. However, it requires a lot of hard work that can make a lasting difference in the well-being of the body.

Many critics have said in their quote that the keto diet can never be healthy because extra fat is taken here. They think fat is the only cause of harm to the body so it is not safe. In conventional society, it is called cholesterol or fat unhygienic. But in fact, fat is a very important mineral for good health. In this diet plan, you can get a lot of fat from healthy sources like red meat, different types of seeds like cherries, palm oil, coconut oil, eggs, butter, fish, nuts, avocado, etc.

Due to the widespread discussion of the ketogenic diet, many critics are reluctant to give accurate information on the subject. In this article, you will get a clear idea about the ketogenic diet and some of its myths.

Keto Diet: Most people are unaware of the Keto diet. The key principle of the keto diet is that it uses fat as a fuel to reduce excess body weight and is interested in eating low carbohydrate foods. The body gradually reduces the number of carbs and replenishes them with fat.

Myth 1: You can eat any type of fat in the diet plan.
Fact: Eat any healthy fats while on the keto diet and do not take saturated fats if you want to stay fit. Eat a diet rich in fiber and eat a certain amount of fat every day.

Myth 2: The main purpose of the Keto diet is to lose weight fast
Fact: In addition to weight loss, the keto diet does a lot of work. Some of them are controlling blood sugar levels, controlling hormones, ensuring intestinal protection, increasing physical function, and so on.

Myth 3: You don't need any practice
Fact: You need to do some exercise when you are on a diet. You must follow some rules while being in the middle of the diet plan. Ensure regular exercise and moderate diet to lose weight fast and. Your body may need carbs during exercise so try to take a certain

amount of carbs.

Myth 4: Muscle mass will decrease a lot
Fact: For those who are on a keto diet to increase energy, it will have the opposite effect. They can increase muscle strength if they want through exercise during the diet.

Myth 5: Feeling tired during the diet
Fact: It is normal to feel tired during the diet, but gradually the fatigue subsides. In many cases, this fatigue does not appear, but if something is noticed, it does not last more than a week at most. The diet is usually short-lived.

Myth 6: There is no scientific basis for dieting
Fact: Diet usually depends on your physical condition and how long you can continue this diet. However, in many cases, as a result of research, science has supported the ketogenic diet. The keto diet was initially introduced to treat epilepsy, which was considered successful. Besides, diet helps in weight loss and staying healthy.

Myth 7: Rich in protein and fat
Fact: The diet is never high in protein and fat. Nutrients are divided based on micronutrients. These diets include moderate amounts of protein, high fat, and low carbs as needed.

Myth 8: Preventing the cause of heart attack
Fact: The keto diet strengthens the intake of saturated fat which prevents heart attacks. There is also control over the number of blood components due to having fewer carbs.

All in all this diet helps to protect your health and improve fitness. Before you start the diet, you must notice its myths and know well about it. There is a lot of evidence-based information available on various websites. There is also a lot of information about the keto diet on our website that is important to start your diet. As the keto diet has many far-reaching benefits, it has become a very popular diet method in a few years. Check out other articles on this topic on our website to get additional information about the keto diet.

Going Keto: Why It's Good For You

Data from the past few years show that the keto diet has been very effective and health-promoting for several reasons. The Quito Diet not only works for weight loss, but it also increases physical fitness for daily work which is a great way. For those who are trying to lose weight fast with the Keto diet, it is not just a diet, it is a way to increase the quality of life. Just as quick results can be obtained during this diet, so too must it be accomplished with some determination and commitment. It is never an easy task; it must bring some changes in daily life.

Many people think that the Quito diet is not for everyone. Although the Quito Diet can change people's quality of life, some people do not want to be a part of it. It is a common practice among us that eating fatty foods increases bodyweight so to lose weight we need to avoid fatty foods which is difficult for us. But there is a widespread practice of eating fat in the Keto diet. This is why they are skeptical of losing weight during this keto diet and they never accept that it has benefits.

Many people have questions about how the Keto diet started. Rollin Woodyatt, an endocrinologist, is thought to have discovered three water-soluble nutrients in 1921: Acetoacetate, B-hydroxybutyrate, and Accenture. He noticed that if a person ate a diet high in fat and low in carbohydrates, his body produced these three nutrients that are effective for a fast diet. It is said that in the same year a man named Russell Wilder named it the ketogenic diet. There has been a widespread response to this great success among young children in the treatment of epilepsy. Due to the progress of treatment, there are many better medical systems instead.

There are many types of diet lists in the Keto diet that can be followed to get results very quickly. The worst experience in the keto diet is keto flu which is often called carb flu. Many times you have to face these problems due to not following the rules of the Keto diet properly. The process by which the human body absorbs energy from glucose is called keto flu, and it is a natural process.

People with keto flu usually experience some serious problems such as severe migraines, restlessness, nausea, shortness of breath, and insomnia. People who think that keto diet are not possible to do these things at the beginning of the Keto diet, so give up this diet; they must make a wrong decision. It should be kept in mind that everyone who starts a keto diet has some unwanted problems like this. If you can get through the first few days of the keto diet, you have had the hardest time. We have mentioned some common steps in this article to start meditation; you can follow them if you want. Some of the notable ones are getting plenty of sleep, eating meat, eating bone broth, taking electrolyte supplements, etc. If you have keto flu, you can take normal food, there is no obstacle in it, but to get protection from it, you must follow some rules.

Normally, when a person eats food, he has a lot of carbohydrates in his diet and the body converts the carbohydrate-rich food into useful glucose according to his needs. Glucose is said to be the main source of the proper functioning of the body. But the amount of carbohydrates in the keto diet is very low so the body has to use any other energy to run smoothly. The body absorbs this energy from fats, which convert fatty acids into ketones.

The percentage of nutrients that should be in the middle of an ideal keto diet is 70-80% fat, 20-25% protein, 5-10% carbohydrate. Foods that contain this amount of nutrients in the keto diet are considered ideal for the keto diet.

You must not eat more than 20 grams of carbs a day while on a ketogenic diet. For a better experience, you can take fewer carbohydrates if you want with some normal symptoms. Ketosis begins when the body is completely dependent on fatty foods. Within the first few days of starting this diet, the body begins to be deficient in internal fatty acids and carbs, and at this time the body is made fit to absorb fat. Fat has many benefits in increasing performance. Excess ketosis can be dangerous for diabetics. On the other hand, the keto diet can be very beneficial for diabetics.

The most challenging part of the keto diet is eating low carbs. Among many foods, it is very troublesome to control. However, it is essential to take healthy fats in this diet. The amount of non-vegetarian food can be taken as it controls the level of diet. Starchy foods must be avoided. Milk and artificial sweeteners can also cause problems. All in all, to live a healthy life, you must follow some rules that make the keto diet much easier.

Keto Dieting? Here Are 10 Foods You Must Have In Your Kitchen

The keto diet is a very commonly suitable and successful diet plan for rapid weight loss and physical fitness. The Keto Diet is currently one of the most popular health supplements through which you can get the nutrients your body needs. If the amount of internal ketosis in your body is 0.5 mmol/L, then you must be in the middle of the keto diet. This diet includes all nutritious foods. If you do not meet all the requirements of the keto diet then you are on the list of low carbohydrate foods which are not included in the keto diet.

In the event of such a physical condition, it is necessary to eat as few carbohydrate foods as possible to maintain a diet in the Keto diet. However, it should be noted that if there is any change in your physical condition, i.e. overall weight and health loss and you feel weak, then you must add nutritious food to the keto diet.

A ketogenic diet uses low carbohydrate and high-fat nutrients to help reduce the amount of internal fat in the body instead of glucose. Many are familiar with the Atkins diet where there are no restrictions on carbohydrate foods but there are considerable limitations between carbohydrate foods in the Keto diet. There are many hotels and restaurants around us where most of the food contains carbohydrates which is very tasty and fun. Avoiding these processed foods during a Keto diet plan can be a bit challenging but there must be some plans that can be adopted instead of these foods.

Before starting this diet, you must make a list of foods so that you are not attracted to delicious food. You also need to make a list of

snacks along with the food list every time so that there are fewer
amounts of carbohydrates. If you want, you can take the help of the
Keto Diet Plan from various online journals and websites. You
follow the Keto lifestyle, choose the desired diet, and stay healthy.

There are some main foods in the keto diet that can be left
incomplete without the keto diet. When making a food list, keep in
mind that heavy cream foods have been legalized in the Keto diet,
meaning fat foods can be included in this diet plan. Be sure to
include the following foods in your Keto diet plan. Below is a
shortlist of 10 ketogenic diet foods:

Eggs: If you like egg dishes, there are many snacks including boiled
egg portions, quiches, omelets, low carbohydrate pizza crust. If you
like to put eggs on the food menu, then of course the Quito Diet has
the potential to be a great success in your diet plan.

Bacon: There is no reason to take bacon with food. Bacon helps to
increase physical fitness and performance. Burger topper, salad
garnish, and bacon can be taken during breakfast. However, bread
should not be eaten in the middle of this type of food because bread
contains a lot of carbohydrates. Mayo can be eaten with Tossed and
you should try to take BLT along with it.

Cream cheese: It is not a barrier to eating fatty foods as it is included
in the keto diet. That's why cream cheese recipes include sweets,
main dishes, pizza crusts, and dozens of other recipes that are much
healthier. In the case of the Keto diet, it is believed that the amount
of internal fat in the body does not increase but decreases when you
exercise by consuming fat.

Shredded cheese: In a bowl, spread the sliced cheese over the taco
meat. Also, shredded cheese can be eaten with enchiladas, low
carbohydrate pizzas, salad toppers, tortilla chips in the microwave,
etc. Shredded cheese is one of the foods in the Keto diet plan that
helps to replenish physical loss and increase energy.

Lots of spinach and romaine: Green vegetables are attached to
almost all diets because these foods help to bring success to the diet

plan quickly and compensate for the loss. In the case of quick meals such as salads can be made very easily and in less time. This type of food is very useful for temporary hunger. Vegetables that can be eaten raw, that are vegetables that are eaten through salads, give many effective results during the diet.

EZ-Liquid Sweets: A few drops of this liquid can be used instead of sugar in sweets. Sweet foods should not be taken at all during the diet plan but they can be used instead of sugar directly. While this healthy liquid can make food taste sweet like sugar, it does not affect the diet. This liquid is natural, healthy, and easy to use. There are no physical side effects so it is safe.

Cauliflower: Cauliflower is another healthy food in the Quito diet. These low-carbohydrate vegetables are a must-have during your diet. Baked and tossed cauliflower and potatoes in olive oil can be eaten in moderation instead of rice. Keto pizza crusts, low carb foods and other foods made with cauliflower can be the most consumed without any change in diet. Cauliflower helps in controlling excess body fat or cholesterol.

Frozen Chicken: There is a tendency to eat a lot of non-vegetarian food in the Keto diet. In the Keto diet, it is believed that non-vegetarian foods are only effective in increasing visual energy, which does not cause any harm to the body. Chicken can be fried by mixing it with low carbohydrate vegetables. Even if it is fried mixed with garlic sauce, it is suitable to eat in the diet of Keto diet.

Ground beef: According to the keto diet, a large burger can be taken to make beef dishes and it can be used with everything from mushrooms to cheese, chopped onions, low-tortilla foods, lettuce, sour cream, avocado, etc.

Almonds: Almonds can be eaten in the Quito diet for breakfast as a healthy and tasty food. Almonds are useful to eat during the diet. Vinegar, salt, coconut, habanero, etc. can also be eaten in the list of snacks.

The Keto Diet is an interesting and versatile way to lose weight fast.

You can store these 10 foods in the fridge so that you can eat them for many days. You can also eat some of these delicious snacks. You can visit other pages, blogs, or websites of the Ketogenesis Diet to get more healthcare tips. You can contact us to get any other information.

Is Your Keto Diet Clean or Dirty

The ketogenic diet has recently gained immense popularity due to its benefits through a high-fat and low carbs diet. Many people follow this type of diet plan to control diabetes and lose weight fast. There are two types of diets, clean and dirty, but the difference between them is not particularly noticeable. So you can learn more about the two parts of the keto diet here. This article is about the difference between a clean and dirty keto diet.

Clean Keto Diet: A clean keto diet usually refers to nutritious foods that are of good quality and traditional. The Clean keto diet contains a certain proportion of nutrients. This diet should include at least 75% of the total daily calorie high fat intake, healthy protein should be 15-220% of the total calories and carbs should be 50 grams.

Dirty Keto Diet: On the other hand, the amount of fat in the dirty keto diet is high and the amount of carbs is relatively low. However, the sources of ingredients in the dirty keto diet are not nutritious in most cases. With this diet, you can achieve the benefits of the keto diet and ketosis. However, in this case, eating all these unhealthy foods can increase the risk of disease in your body and some useful nutrients can be omitted.

Like the Keto diet tips, the CrossFit diet also mentions diet programs mainly for athletes. Even if you follow the paleo regimen or keto diet plan, there are some bad ways and some good ways. A complete diet plan is not known by just one name. If the foods you are taking according to the diet plan are of low quality, then they will do more harm than good to you, that is, it will be harmful to your health. In this article, we will discuss the types of ketosis in the keto diet. To increase ketones in your body, you have to take food according to the keto diet plan.

According to the keto diet plan, high fat intake results in the production of ketone by the liver. This process begins with a regular and adequate intake of protein and low carbohydrates. The internal functions of the body are properly regulated through the use of energy derived from ketones. In other words, fat is used to manage the body's biological functions through the keto diet. Your body goes into a state of ketosis only when the body starts producing ketones. As long as you continue to eat according to the ketogenic diet, your body will continue to expend excess fat.

At this stage of the article, clean keto diet and dirty keto diet have been discussed. Since carbohydrate-rich foods are rarely included in such diet plans, low-carb vegetables, seafood, or a variety of sugars may be part of the national diet. However, in the middle of this diet plan, you should refrain from eating commercially supplied fast food like fish, meat, or burgers. If you eat only carbs, you must include a dirty keto diet which is a major obstacle to good health.

During this keto diet plan, we advise you to stay away from all kinds of preservative foods. These preserved foods are harmful to any diet and can harm your health. Once the food is basic and clean, it can work well for any diet. Usually, the detoxifying process is in the middle of the keto diet. So you must keep in mind that if you add toxins through food, it will not help your health and liver.

Try to eat fresh green and fiber-rich vegetables regularly to manage the keto diet properly. The more you try to eat these foods, the better for your health. Eating fresh vegetables is good for health and enhances the taste of more foods. Choose healthy sources of fatty foods. These may include coconut oil, avocados, olive oil, organic fructose, etc. Many of these foods are marked as non-inflammatory and many of them cause inflammation in the stomach. One of them is dairy food.

When running a clean keto diet, remember to eat small amounts of good carbohydrates and fats. However, while doing the keto diet, you must drink plenty of pure water which helps in the proper development of the organs and digestion of food. Always try to abstain from the dirty keto diet. The diet lists of this type of keto diet are obtained from low-quality and unhealthy sources which are different from the clean keto diet.

A healthy keto diet suggests nutritious and high-quality fatty foods. The dirty version pays more attention to preservative foods. According to the clean keto diet, it is recommended to eat starch-free vegetables like asparagus, broccoli, kale, and spinach, but the dirty keto diet can eat fewer vegetables and have relatively high sodium content in their diet. It is generally said that for long-term health one should eliminate dirty keto diet and follow a clean keto diet to reduce the risk of malnutrition and disease.

All about Intermittent Fasting

Intermittent fasting refers to the long-term intake of dietary foods. Once you start the diet, there is no need to follow it for life. There are many types of diets available during Ramadan that is as healthy as diet plans. The topic of maintaining good health and physical fitness has now become very important and popular in a scientific way.

Intermittent Fasting: Naturally, many people have been avoiding food voluntarily during periods or fasting for ages. Many people do intermittent fasting considering the improvement of health. In almost every diet, it is strictly forbidden to eat for a certain period and it does not matter what food you eat during this time. One or two days per week, the most popular intermittent fasting at present, is too fast for a certain time every day. It is very beneficial for the body to take a break or fast between regular meals.

From the experience of the ancestors who went hunting, it is easy to understand how important it is to take food at regular intervals.

These eating habits start from old age and help in bodybuilding and longevity. It can be seen that this intermittent fasting routine works against daily eating habits and culture but less food should be taken during dinner, lunch, snacks, and snacks scientifically. So the intermittent fasting diet has gained popularity as an alternative to following this diet. This article mentions two myths related to this starvation.

Myth 1: You must eat on time every day. This common practice in our society is not only designed to promote improved health, it was first adopted in general and later accepted as ideal as it provides very good feedback. Eating three meals a day is not only scientific but also seen in the context of various studies which are best for health. Also eating the same amount of calories per day is good for bodybuilding. However, it will be better when a person consumes a certain amount of food regularly for dieting because nothing irregular is harmful to health.

Myth 2: You must have a regular breakfast. This is a very important meal for a healthy start to the day. There are many myths about breakfast that are completely unfounded. Having a regular breakfast helps normalize metabolism and increases daily performance. Over a long period, it has been proven that regular breakfast intake did not cause any significant problems in the metabolic process, and as a result, there was no change between dinner and lunch but some unusual changes can be noticed if breakfast is not eaten properly. Breakfast is a very important meal - it can either make or break your day.

Different parts of intermittent fasting: There are different types of intermittent fasting and each has its specific benefits. It is divided into different parts based on the proportion of food. Different intermittent fasting has different efficacy and benefits, it is important to decide which of them is best for you. The two most common types of intermittent fasting are modified fasting and time-limited eating. Some of them are given below:

1. Alternate day fasting: During this processing can triglyceride or fat, control blood cholesterol, and lose weight very quickly. It also

improves the normal flow of blood through this plan. However, the main problem with this fasting is that it becomes relatively difficult to follow this rule during the days of Ramadan.

2. Diet of Modified Fasting: Modified fasting gives a special protocol for programmed fasting which allows taking some calorie-rich food on fasting days. You need to consume 20-25% more calories during fasting than the total calories of a normal day, which means you will consume one-fourth more calories than any other day. The 5: 2 ratios between these diets represent the ratio of meals to normal days and fasting days. In the middle of the week, you will take one-fourth of the amount of food you take every 5 days for the next 2 days.

This diet can be of great help in controlling inflammation, lipids, blood sugar, and bodybuilding. However, going through this intermittent fasting process to burn fat increases the protein level in the body comparatively most of the time which causes uncomfortable situations. Doing this fasting ratio of 5: 2 helps to control blood sugar and reduce hunger hormones. However, there are some negative reactions at the beginning of this fasting, such as some annoyance, low energy, loss of appetite, etc. However, it has some positive changes such as normal mood, improved self-confidence, less fatigue, less anger, etc.

3. Time-restricted feeding: If you know someone who is fasting non-stop, their problems are time-restricted feeding. It is a kind of non-stop fasting process that allows you to take in calories in a very short period and suggest fasting the rest of the time. The time between days between these protocols is not so important that you do not eat continuously. The more time you spend in a day without eating, the better.

Intermittent fasting is one of the easiest ways of time-restricted feeding. It is best to follow these rules in addition to your sleep schedule and daily activities that help manage metabolic functions. Maintaining health benefits is a great way to build a body and lose weight fast. Intermittent fasting is done to protect against some deadly harmful diseases like fatty liver disease, high insulin levels, body weight gain, etc.

Due to the commitment and easy application of time-restricted feeding, it can be effective in preventing chronic diseases and weight loss. Foods that do not contain calories or are low in calories can be taken during fasting. According to many, black coffee during fasting can reduce appetite. Sometimes fasting has many long-term benefits. Some of the significant benefits of fasting are highlighted below:

Applicable to human which are -
- Lose weight fast
- Improving blood lipid markers is like cholesterol
- Reduces physical inflammation
- Confidence increases and stress decreases
- Possesses improved mood

Applicable to animals which are-
- Reduces body fat
- Decreasing the levels of leptin which is known as appetite hormone
- Improves insulin levels
- Prevents physical inflammation, fatty liver disease, obesity
- By longevity

All in all, intermittent fasting is very important for keeping the body healthy which is very popular nowadays. This will help you lose weight very quickly and reduce excess body fat. Intermittent fasting is done to protect against many diseases which is a major obstacle in consuming extra calories. Through this intermittent fasting, one can easily return to his normal life. You will find many more detailed ideas about this on our website. Don't hesitate to ask us if you have any questions or concerns.

Fasting for Weight Loss – Learn How To Lose Weight Quickly By Doing THIS!

Fasting is usually used in the hope of gaining spiritual meditation or faith in a religion. In many cases, fasting is seen as a protest against any political opinion to get the demand. In between fasts, one should abstain from any kind of drink or food for a certain period. However, many people nowadays fast to remove harmful toxins from their bodies or to lose weight.

Fasting is a very popular weight loss program that is different from every diet. Some fasts allow only liquid food such as tea, fruit juice, water, etc. Many fasts keep the calorie intake right without eating. You must keep in mind how healthy or effective your fasting is for your body to lose weight. Here are some tips to help you lose weight fast and here are some of the notable ones:

• Decide to do intermittent fasting from time to time. Usually take a certain amount of food on days other than fasting.
• During fasting, you must consume an adequate amount of calories. Eat healthy fats, complex carbohydrates, and reduced protein so that your body can provide the energy it needs during fasting.
• Try to reduce physical activity as much as possible during fasting. Excessive exercise can be harmful to your body which also prevents you from fasting.
• Take care of your body and find a little way that is good and beneficial for your body. If for some reason you can't concentrate on fasting, are tired or sick, and have headaches, then fasting will not be beneficial for you.
• Choose a specific period to fast during the diet. Before starting fasting, you must take the advice of a doctor that there is no health risk if you fast.

The easiest and fastest way to lose weight is to exercise daily. One can complete daily physical exercise through cycling, swimming, walking, running, etc. These enjoyable and easy things can be done to lose weight fast. During fasting, you must refrain from any hard work and it is important to remember.

Various reasons for fasting: When you fast for a certain period to create a detoxifying state in your body, your physical condition goes into ketosis. So, burning excess fat to lose weight can cause ketosis because carbohydrates are not burned to provide energy. This causes detoxification in the body because most of the body's fats contain toxins. It is important to fast before surgery, before checking cholesterol levels, before diagnosing blood sugar levels, and for spiritual or religious purposes. Fasting is also effective in treating low blood pressure, eczema, psoriasis, Crohn's disease, ulcerative colitis, lupus, heart disease, arthritis, and depression. Certain calorie-restricted diets help a person to prolong life. Periodic fasting and moderate eating habits help a person to live a healthy life. Fasting also helps in dealing with frustration and stress.

There are several major benefits to fasting, and each one is closely related to the other. Fasting can complement each other as well as improve your health. Below are the two main ways of fasting:

• Juice or water fasting: Only liquid juice or water can be consumed during this fast. Green vegetables and fresh fruits can be taken during this fast. These provide essential nutrients, as well as help, keep the body healthy.
• Endless fasting: This method involves fasting regularly and taking certain foods. Such fasting can be done almost every day of the week.

During fasting, the metabolic rate is slow so it helps to reduce appetite. Glycogen can be used to keep the body functioning on the first day of fasting. Naturally, fat is needed when the body does not get enough carbohydrates to maintain its performance. Gradually the protein is converted to glucose instead of carbohydrates.

Importance of fasting for weight loss: Fasting is safe for people who consume adequate amounts of fluids. Fasting is not safe for those with poor immune function, cardiac arrhythmia, diabetes, kidney or liver problems, malnutrition, etc.

Advantages of fasting: Fasting has anti-aging effects on the skin and helps to control appetite. Fasting helps to create new brain cells and increase density. It also helps to make healthy changes in lifestyle and diet.

Disadvantages of fasting: Sudden low-calorie intake can lower BMR and increase health risks. Lack of nutrients, minerals, and vitamins needed to keep the body healthy. Excessive diet plans and fasting can lead to health problems and need urgent treatment.

Fasting for weight loss is safe only when it is done moderately and correctly. The main advantage of fasting is that it works for rapid weight loss and helps reduce appetite. Fasting helps you to be confident and can increase physical performance. The easiest way to lose weight permanently is to live without food at a certain time called fasting. As a result of fasting, the internal activities of the body get a chance to work well again and as a result, many diseases are cured. Fasting also helps you change your thinking and live a healthier life.

Fasting to Burn Fat

There are many benefits to fasting for those who are already in the middle of fasting. There are many benefits to fasting and it should be enjoyed by all but one must be amid a healthy diet and healthy lifestyle. If you try too fast to lose weight and it fails, then the whole effort will be in vain. You can collect a lot of information about fasting from our website. We are hopeful that we will be able to give you more information than you wanted.

However, keep in mind that the benefits of fasting are never the same for everyone and in many cases the response is different. In this case, the response and conditions of the two types of fasting may be different. So never compare your results with anyone while fasting, but the most important thing here is how your soul, mind, and body can feel the positive change.

Different types of fasting: There are different ways to fast. There are various ways in which fasting is usually practiced. Below is a brief discussion of some kinds of fasting:

Complete fast: between complete fast, you can drink one glass of hot water with lemon juice and one glass of normal temperature mineral water at regular intervals. Lemon juice is eaten with hot water to protect the stomach from acidity and lemon juice with hot water also works for rapid weight loss. Also if one goes to gain extra energy if needed, one can eat it by mixing some honey with lemon juice. Gentle coconut water can also be taken during this fast.

Banana-Milk Diet: This type of diet includes a banana and a cup of skimmed milk two to three times a day. At the same time, lemon juice and honey can be taken for drinking light hot water. The milk banana diet is considered to be the most effective and readily available.

Fruit diet: In this diet, a person can eat only fruit juice and fruits. Lemon juice can be eaten with hot water during this fast. However, the fasting of this fruit should not be done for more than 6-7 days as it may weaken the body. Excessive fasting of fruits can also lead to a deficiency of essential amino acids and enzymes in the body. Naturally, a fruit diet is effective for losing excess weight so it is very popular nowadays.

Vegetables and fruits: Fresh fruits, steamed or cooked vegetables can be included in this type of diet. However, in the middle of this diet plan, you must refrain from eating extra salt. The duration of this diet plan cannot be more than 6-7 days as more than this can lead to physical complications.

Traditional fast: Traditional fasts are usually done at certain times of the year and at this time some light meals can be taken once a day. These foods may contain little fat, sugar, and salt. However, no one takes to juice, tea, vegetables, or fruits as the main food during this fast. At the end of the day, lemon juice can be eaten with hot water which is effective for rapid weight loss. This kind of fast can be observed on a specific day of the Arabic month, the day of the full moon, or the occasion of any puja.

Water fast: You can fast continuously for 1-40 days between these water fasts. At this time, try to drink more than 2 liters of water per day on average. Significant changes can be noticed in the next 30 days after 10 days have elapsed between these fasts. If your metabolic process is much faster than water fasting becomes much harder for you. Fasting in water can be very effective in removing toxins and contaminants from the body quickly. Water fasting can work against cancer which is more effective than any juice fasting. Water fasting also helps to clean severely damaged and damaged tissues. Fasting on water reduces your peace of mind and stress and normalizes your quality of life. Many people suggest that you should eat more fresh fruits, vegetables, and fruit juices in the first few days before starting fasting to reduce the detoxification of the body during fasting. Fasting with water and juice is one of the best ways to gain physical fitness and increase performance.

Juice fast: fasting juice is more effective and healthy than any other fast. This fasting allows for the removal of toxins called toxins from the body to greatly improve health and maintain good health. One of the benefits of this diet is that you can continue to lead a normal life because you are getting enough nutrients from fruit juices. Fruit juice can usually work to smooth the skin as well as solve many physical complications. Also fasting fruit juice fills the deficiency of nutrients in the body. Fruit juice works to provide energy to the body quickly. An adequate amount of calories, photochemical, antioxidants, living enzymes, minerals, vitamins, etc. can be filled through fruit juice. Fruit fasting also works for the well-being of the mind and the protection of strong physical health.

All in all, fasting plays a very important role in protecting health. Just as fasting is beneficial for rapid weight loss, so is fasting for good health. Fasting relieves many physical complications and disabilities which are often a matter of medicine or any other means. By fasting, a person can perform normal activities in his daily life very well without any side effects. On the other hand, fasting can reduce excess body fat quickly, which is one of the reasons for many fatal diseases.

Tips for Fasting Success

Many people are willing to improve their health and lose weight but they do not know how to start with fasting. Again they do not get full support from friends or family when they start by fasting because they do not have full knowledge about the benefits of fasting. Again, there are many people whose physical condition is not healthy for this doctor does not allow it. You must take the advice of a doctor considering your physical condition.

The point to be made here is that no one can know better about your physical condition more than you. Being overweight can lead to diabetes, heart attack, and other health risks, and these are important enough to disrupt someone's normal quality of life. Increasing body weight greatly reduces immunity. If you want, you can find out more about this from various websites on the internet or you can visit the articles on our website.

There are many effective and healthier ways you can fast water for fast success. You can choose any day of the week for this fast. You can fast for 8, 12, or 24 hours a day if you want to lose weight fast and feel the positive change. This is a very easy and fast way to lose weight so it is very popular nowadays.

Choose a fasting strategy or diet plan based on your body condition that will not have any detrimental effects on your body and you will be able to stay fit. Water fasting can be difficult but effective for you if you are new to fasting. So do not start the diet with any fasting at the beginning that may cause you frustration.

However, if you have to fast while following some traditional rituals, you must take the advice of a doctor. If your doctor's advice is against fasting, be sure to ask him or her for a minimum period. Sometimes you can fast for eight hours or less a day. Be sure to let the doctor know that you are not following a crash diet. You need to make some changes in your total eating habits. Decide to fast base on the physical condition and doctor's advice after changing the diet.

Fasting is one of the ways to protect health that is natural and proven. Instead of fasting, there are many types of medicines available in the markets that help in rapid weight loss. It is better not to take these medicines because these medicines have many side effects which are harmful to health. There must be some effort to get the most feedback from any fast. Eating sweets during fasting should be completely avoided and fresh and fresh fruits or vegetables should be taken in large quantities.

During fasting, you can eat organically grown vegetables or fruits which reduce the deficiency of nutrients in the body and keeps the body functioning. On the other hand, if you want to fast water then you must drink good quality and adequate amount of water. For this, the water must be filtered and purified. If you don't have the opportunity to filter the water, you can boil it before drinking it.

Decaffeinated green tea works as a great supplement to quench hunger and provide the necessary energy during fasting. But to be successful in fasting, you must follow certain rules. However, the main thing to be successful in fasting is to do regular and regular physical exercise. Regular exercise works against the accumulation of excess body fat and keeps the body and mind healthy. The results of fasting may vary from person to person. For some people, the results are quick to reveal while for others it becomes a matter of time. Try to fast from time to time and notice the significant differences that will inspire you for fasting.

Prepare yourself about a week before breaking the fast, which is very important to keep the body healthy. If you are not prepared in advance about this fast, this excess appetite can cause severe damage to your intestines and cause great discomfort. You can learn more about the importance of fasting from various websites. Be sure to be aware when the fasting period is over because you have experienced much great rejuvenation and recovery. After fasting, very low fat and low-fat foods such as milk, sodas, alcohol, additives, sugars, carbohydrates can be taken in very small amounts.

Fasting should be the main and important way to live a healthy life. If you know the benefits of fasting, you will be committed to ending the fast with self-satisfaction and enjoyment. Fasting is an ingredient that helps you change your eating habits by following a set of rules. Fasting has many benefits due to its popularity and success rate.

Bodyweight Exercise for Losing Weight

Regularly individuals commit errors with regards to bodyweight work out. They see ads on TV where they see their famous people embracing how these activities have assisted them with losing abundance fat off their bodies and tone up their body. Taking a gander at these advertisements, many feel that bodyweight practices are very straight ward and that they are liberated from any danger. Actually, on the chance that you don't practice as expected, the odds are that you will hurt yourself gravely. Numerous projects will assist you with doing weight practices cautiously. These are planned by experts who have just tried the viability of the projects and realize that whenever done appropriately it can likewise work for you.

At the point when you are simply beginning your program, it is better that you start your preparation with a bodyweight just program so you can take it overall quite simple, without the dread of harming yourself in the deal. There are programs with various that centers around dealing with the various territories of your body. It is proposed that you play it safe to lessen the odds of injury. Guarantee that you are not with regards to your bodyweight schedule.

Since an appropriately planned bodyweight routine can be very demanding, it is significant that you practice alert while working out. Significantly, you release up before starting your activities and after finishing, permit your body to chill off effectively. Heating up and chilling off is an extremely essential piece of any bodyweight practices program. The heating up measure helps in the jump-starting system while the chilling off causes your body to return to the typical state.

Another part of bodyweight practices is that the vast majority feel that it is straightforward and simple. Be that as it may, it is not accurate and requires a lot of consideration and care while doing the activities. You must hit the nail on the head without fail, else you can get harmed. Even though bodyweight practices are among the most un-unsafe of activities, still you need to show alert and not be imprudent while working out. It is proposed that you experience a delineated guide or purchase a video showing you the correct. This is one method of accomplishing your objective without really harming yourself all the while.

There are numerous individuals who in their journey to accomplish results rapidly, over work out. These individuals don't understand the effect it will have on their bodies. It is essential to accomplish results yet it ought to be in an orderly way. Increment your practicing routine however it does slowly so your body can become acclimated to it. Else, you risk harming yourself all the while. It is proposed that you increment the reiterations dynamically in your everyday exercise so your body becomes acclimated to it and it additionally encourages you tightens up your body at an agreeable speed. Throughout some undefined time frame, you can build the speed just as the trouble levels in your bodyweight practicing a routine with the goal that you will accomplish the ideal outcomes rapidly. In this case, ensure that you practice the funametic alert and increment the trouble levels just when you are agreeable.

Bodyweight practices are likewise frequently joined into stop-and-go aerobic exercise (HIIT), which Tom said "is an amazingly proficient approach to diminish muscle versus fat, "and develop fortitude. You can do HIIT with both cardio and strength preparing, and because HIIT exercises are commonly beautiful short (you can just keep up max-exertion work for such a long time!), you should frequently be possible quickly or less. The comfort and low-time responsibility make bodyweight HIIT circuits simpler to stay with than weightlifting for a great many people.

That implies, indeed, you can get thinner doing bodyweight works out. As you develop your wellness and begin to consume fat, however, you'll need to discover approaches to build the trouble of your moves. Reformist over-burden, a term generally utilized with weightlifting, applies to bodyweight exercise too: you need to expand the weight you're lifting to continue to challenge your muscles and body.

So, how would you increment the power of a bodyweight exercise without moving to loads? Many people suggested adding plyometric (bouncing) moves as a "basic approach to build the force and up the calorie consume." This may mean you tread normal bodyweight squats with hop squats, customary rushes with hopping jumps, or even push-ups with plyometric push-ups. These moves are intended to be testing, so it's fine to require some investment developing to them. Attempt this ploy circuit when you're prepared to reduce bodyweight.

At long last, you ought to comprehend that a bodyweight practices routine is intended to assist you with accomplishing the greatest advantage via a solid and fit body. You presently don't need to spend heaps of cash on going to exercise centers and health clubs.

3 Ways in Which You Can Optimize the Use of Bodyweight Exercise

Maintaining body weight and exercising regularly is very important for maintaining physical fitness. There should be some variation between bodyweight exercise programs that make daily exercise fun. Some people do not like bodyweight programs and many people do regular bodyweight programs just to keep fit. This is why some people think that bodyweight maintenance programs are very necessary to maintain the level of physical fitness and performance but many do not think so.

However, according to most experts, physical fitness is not the only way to maintain physical fitness, it is necessary to do some extra curriculum activities. There must be active participation in maintaining a good balance between physical training programs. In this article, we have divided bodyweight exercise into three parts through which you will get a clear idea about body fitness. From beginners to experienced weightlifters, everyone exercises for exercise. But experienced bodybuilders only do bodyweight exercise. In this article, three types of bodyweight exercises are discussed below:

Bodyweight exercise for beginners: Commercial gym is usually suggested for any strength training. To increase cardiorespiratory endurance to exercise in a commercial gym, you are usually asked to use cardio equipment like a machine. This is of course a general course to increase bodyweight. However, most gyms recommend taking this type of training to increase cardio performance and keep breathing. Of course, this cardio is a very difficult exercise for newcomers, but it is fun to get used to it in a few days. Even if a beginner has no previous experience, he can do all these bodyweight exercises with the help of machines to maintain his physical fitness.

You can easily increase your physical stimulation through physical training which improves the quality of life. Bodyweight exercise is a very reasonable place for beginners. This is because most beginners get lost and inactive due to a lack of proper guidelines. For a beginner, it is important to think about how to perform the exercise without any physical resistance. So before starting the exercise, you have to try the good performance of bodyweight. Once you have mastered all the bodyweight techniques, exercise is improved and prevention is added.

Bodyweight Exercise Techniques for Experienced Weightlifters: Many skilled and experienced people find bodyweight exercise ineffective and neglect physical training. They use a variety of illegal training methods while ignoring these bodyweight methods. Physical fitness training programs can be used to tackle any challenging task and increase performance in sports. These will usually be managed through the movement and effective control of your body. Bodyweight exercise is the best way to train the body to control and move properly. Some of the techniques of bodyweight exercise include pushups. If you can do pushups you can try more to increase the extra strength. You will be able to notice some specific improvements and physical changes through training. Even if you are an experienced weightlifter, you need to practice it regularly.

Bodyweight exercise for crowd only: This article supports bodyweight exercise but not exclusively. Physical fitness programs are used exclusively between different bodyweight exercises. Through this type of training only a bodybuilder can move towards the excellence of his fitness but success depends on him. It must be remembered that yoga exercise must be related to meditation. Again and again, Pilates was developed as a form of rehabilitation for war veterans. Bodyweight training will only teach you some techniques and you will need to apply them.

Balanced bodyweight exercise is important as part of any physical fitness program. For beginners, starting a bodyweight exercise is a good idea. If you are trying to increase your physical fitness, you can practice it to increase your physical fitness. If you are only trying to practice bodyweight, add these with it and diversify your fitness program. Never underestimate bodyweight exercise. Try to use your limitations, abilities, needs, goals, and skills in the right proportions and in the right way in every field of life.

Bodyweight Exercise Program – 2 Things to Avoid If You Want Extraordinary Results

The best way to build a strong physique, burn excess body fat and improve physical fitness is to exercise regularly. Your body weight exercise is a program related to style to improve your health. Never underestimate the easy bodyweight exercises, but you can challenge them to compete among experienced athletes.

If you want to get good feedback from bodyweight exercise, you must follow some strategies. This article contains some bodyweight exercise techniques that you can follow to make your body more capable, burn unwanted body fat and improve physical fitness. Try not to do a bodyweight exercise for your extraordinary success. This can be between any type of bodyweight exercise program or physical training. There are usually some good bodyweight exercises between men and women that they are not interested in learning any other technique until they do. The main problem here is that through such thinking they become more interested in the faded unicorn of bodyweight exercise and spend time.

Almost all of us know that there is no strategy in the bodyweight exercise program that will work in all situations and needs. So it would be foolish to look for such a strategy, so refrain from doing such a thing. For your good performance, you must look at different strategies that will keep you ahead of the subject.

Bodyweight exercise to maintain proper physical fitness: Physical fitness usually increases mental strength, accuracy, agility, coordination, balance, flexibility, speed, cardiorespiratory endurance, and strength. An ideal body weight exercise should have all these qualities through which one can increase his body muscle as well as overall defense. So, all body skills should be ensured by practicing a bodyweight exercise that can be enhanced physical fitness and external beauty. So you need to find a physical program that is effective for bodyweight workouts.

The role of bodyweight exercise in reducing fat: Most people want to burn excess and unwanted body fat which is detrimental to their normal quality of life, so they can take the help of a good bodyweight exercise program. Try practicing calisthenics and body weight with a little rest. This is a better way to burn fat than any other trade mill. So in all your bodyweight exercises, you should add a workout to reduce the most lost fat.

Bodyweight exercise in proportion to size and strength: Excluding some popular techniques, you can become stronger and more experienced only through bodyweight exercises. If the goal of your bodyweight exercise is only to increase muscle size, it is not possible with just this one type of exercise. However, it can be said for sure that there is a special athlete technique to increase the size and strength of the muscles through which the body is used to pump more muscles which is related to physical exercise. Used to increase muscle strength and size as well as burn excess body fat and maintain a fitness workout. The best way to achieve your bodyweight exercise is to practice through a variety of workouts. Of the many exercises, three types of bodyweight exercises are given in this article. One of them is a variety of strong and larger muscle-building techniques to increase physical fitness and try on them. In the same way, you will move towards building artificial muscles, fat and strong muscles without reducing the effectiveness of the workout or getting bored.

Cardiovascular training for energy training isolation: You can see workouts related to cardio training and individual resistance training whenever you go to any gym. Usually, you do resistance exercise at the beginning of your bodyweight exercise and later you can do about 25-30 cardio exercises or jogging exercises.

I don't think there is a problem with this method. But if you want to work with full mental strength, cardiorespiratory endurance, and full strength of the body, you need to take training to master all these things. There are several things that you need to work a little harder to master when practicing bodyweight. Calisthenics and bodyweight exercises allow you to control and attack mental strength, lungs, heart, and all the muscles of the body.

If you want the best results through bodyweight practice, you must take training on these topics. So if you want to get good feedback from bodyweight practice, you need to workout to learn the line between cardio and resistance training. If you follow the methods mentioned in our article, you will be surprised to see the results of bodyweight workouts later. Also, contact us to get any information about bodyweight practice or stay tuned with all the updates on our website.

Five Tips for Getting the Most from Your Bodyweight Exercise

Workout

Bodyweight practices are planned so you can utilize your own "bodyweight" to give the strain and apposition regularly connected with weight preparing gear. Nonetheless, bodyweight practices are not the same as conventional weight preparing in that while it limits explicit regions of your body for developing fortitude and perseverance, despite customary weight preparing strategies it likewise develops fortitude and perseverance all through your entire body.

There are five hints for benefiting as much as possible from the technique for bodyweight work out. To begin with, utilize planned circuits. Second, add cardiovascular activities to your bodyweight practice exercise. Third, to accomplish fat consuming outcomes, separate your activity routine into a few short schedules for the day rather than one long one. Fourth, keep an exercise log. Fifth, change your everyday practice. Try not to allow it to get exhausting, on the off chance that is you would prefer not to do it any longer. I will tell you more five tips.

•   Play with tempo: Hinder squats, pushups, and leg lifts to make them harder-your muscles will invest additional energy under pressure. Accelerate dynamic developments, similar to hikers, board jacks, and high knees, which will prepare your anaerobic framework to assemble more force and light extra calories.
•   Throw in a prop: "Bodyweight" doesn't need to mean no gear-simply, not the stacked kind. Take a stab at raising your feet with a seat in gluten extension and thrusts. The tallness ups the test by expanding the distance your body needs to go against gravity.
•   Move around: Adding horizontal, forward, or in reverse development to any activity (think strolling hands up or venturing feet aside after a board) initiates muscles that may have been simply Chilin. More muscle initiation=better consumption.
•   Refresh the ratio: The more limited your "on" span, the harder you ought to be working. To increase your force, slice down that stretch to 20 or 30 seconds and give yourself the additional opportunity to all the more likely recuperate. Or on the other hand, keep your work span the equivalent and trim your rest time, so your

body stays in the extreme focus, fat-impacting zone.

• Create a combo: Take a move you've done on various occasions (seeing you, squats) and interface an ensuing one (a star bounce, a kick, whatever streams) to it.

Now, I will tell you about coordinated circuits. The international sports Science Association characterizes high-intensity aerobics as a progression of activities, performed consistently, with little rest in the middle. For instance, finishing 30 sit-ups, at that point 30 pushups every one of them in 30 seconds with a 30 rest in the middle would be an illustration of coordinated circuits. Perhaps the most worthwhile parts of planned circuits are their flexibility to your particular objective, accomplishment in a game, or to your wellness level.

Adding cardiovascular activities to your bodyweight practices is significant because it keeps your pulse up just as empowers overall body work out. To fuse cardio schedules in your bodyweight practice routine is to just stroll preceding working out, however, a superior strategy is to utilize a few warm-ups and extending practices in a planned circuit's schedule. For instance, start with steps, add wide-swinging arms, at the point of a bodyweight exercise, and afterward add rushes. The cardio part ought to likewise be restricted on schedule and reiterations.

For both the bodyweight practice and cardiovascular schedules to accomplish the most ideal for consuming outcomes you should split them up into more limited exercise more than once every day. Rather than a complete daily practice for 30 minutes, attempt three ten minutes exercise a day. Attempt this rather than a quick rest at the workplace, you may return restored.

Monitoring your daily schedule, either by composing it in a scratchpad, utilizing a web-based preparing log, bookkeeping page you have made all alone or one of the number books accessible only, for this reason, encourages you in monitoring your occasions, redundancies, individuals accomplishments, objective and development in your bodyweight practice schedule. A preparation log can give you motivating force to contend with yourself or work out accomplice just as certain certification of your advancement.

Ultimately, have a go at different your daily schedule. Take a gander at your preparation record and switch up the bodyweight practices you use consistently. Since there are around 25 standard activities that nearly everybody knows, from fledgling to proficient it is not difficult to one or the other keep to the ones you know the best or to not capitalize on your bodyweight practice directing by adding various activities, changing the weight of opposition.

You can likewise change up your bodyweight practice routine by leasing recordings (don't buy then you utilize a similar one again and again) or ask companions, family, or colleagues to practice with you. Make a point to incorporate those bodyweights and cardio practices you like the best while fluctuating your daily schedule, that way you can do what you like and benefit as much as possible from it.

Indeed, even a ten-moment bodyweight exercise can be successful utilize these tips. By taking advantage of your bodyweight practice exercise you can support your digestion, fabricate muscle, and shape your body without long periods, costly supplies, or exhausting activities you have no interest in.

How to Build Muscle with Bodyweight Exercise

The most widely recognized mix-up made by individuals who try to assemble muscle with bodyweight practices today is they neglect to follow the standards of muscle development and rather perform high reiteration sets of basic activities. For instance, you can't fabricate an amazing chest by doing sets of 30, 50, or even 100 ups as these breaks the standards of muscle development and can just bring about improved solid perseverance.

The number of reps and sets required for body muscle gaining

After very nearly 100 hundred years of experimentation it has been exhibited reliably that the best nearly way to deal with developing muscle size is a standard that contains 4 exercises of 3-4 plans of 6-10 emphases for each muscle. This is the structure that in every practical sense, all master athletes use today and is the very system that Legends, for instance, Arnold Schwarzenegger and Frank Zane used 35 years earlier and that is because it works.

Your body doesn't separate between the check offered through weight planning or your own body and thusly if you follow a comparable number of exercise, sets, and redundancies for building muscle with bodyweight rehearses as you would loads you will get comparable results. So the secret is to reliably grow the difficulty of your bodyweight rehearses so a lot of 6-10 reps are just about as troubling as a movement with burdens would be.

The two ways of gaining more demanding bodyweight exercise The essential strategy used to grow the force of a bodyweight practice and in this manner engage you to keep inside the 6-10 rep range needed for muscle improvement is to change the circumstance of your body fairly to alter the impacts being publicized. For example, in an action, for instance, press-ups you can progress from standard variation to gem, hip, and subsequently panache press up. All of these exercises are more irksome than the previous one and you are hence prepared to use the head of development to make growing degrees of fortitude and muscle. If you consider that in over 20 years of guaranteeing exercise focuses I could check the number of people that can do 10 panache presses ups one hand you can see how with a little inventive psyche you can by and large keep the number of reps inside the 6-10 domain required.

The second procedure for growing the power of bodyweight rehearses is to ceaselessly progress from the two-limbed to extremity type of a movement. In case you take pull-ups, for example, you can progress from standard two arms-ups to negative one arm pull-ups to finally doing one-arm pull-ups. I have never seen any who can do 10 consecutive one-arm pull-ups so remember it is reliably possible to keep the emphasis range in the 6-10 domain expected to manufacture muscle with bodyweight works out.

You should train yourself per week in a certain period
We are completely restricted by time limitations throughout
everybody's life and with work, family, and the overall necessities of
everyday living it is here and difficult to fit in your instructional
courses. Notwithstanding, on the off chance that you need to
construct muscle with bodyweight practices you need to complete 4
meetings each week utilizing a split routine which empowers you to
prepared you to prepare both the top and base piece of your body
two times every week.

Quality of training
It doesn't make any difference what kind of preparing you to do or
how frequently seven days you train, if the power isn't there you are
burning through your time. You can energize muscle development if
you continually make the muscle work more diligently.

The muscle-building Diet
The eating routine you exercise is the main factor for muscle
development and any reasonable person would agree that you will
possibly succeed on the off chance that you observe certain
guidelines.To shield you from conceivable injury your body adjusts
to your activity program by building more muscle so it can adapt
better to the requests you put on it the following time you train. In
any case, nothing can be worked from nothing and your body can
not construct muscle except if you finish it with the supplements it
needs to incorporate the accompanying.

Calories, you need to ensure you devour 500 a greater number of
calories each day than your body would have to keep up your current
weight. Protein, aside from water, muscle is made up essentially of
protein and it follows that to assemble more muscle you need to
burn-through more protein. It is additionally suggested that you eat
just great quality food that eating routine is comprised of 50 % crabs
(chiefly complex ones like earthy colored rice and green vegetables),
25 % protein like lean meat, fish, and eggs, and 25% fats(mainly
monounsaturated and polyunsaturated fats from olive oil, nuts seeds,
and sunflower oil.

If you follow these rules you should build your bodyweight by roughly 1 pound each week. In any case, everyone is exceptional so it isn't projected in stone, and some experiments possibly important to get the correct equilibrium.

Sleep

Rest is the point at which all your hard preparing pays off the fact that it is the point at which you rest that your body fixes itself and makes you greater and more grounded. Attempt to get at any rate 7 or 8 hours rest each night. In the event you be adequately youthful to need to party the entire end of the week, the add late night will not damage you get if you continually party you won't gain as much ground as might somehow be the situation.

Motivation

Inspiration is without question the absolute most significant thing required for building muscle or whatever else throughout everyday life. Despite some other factor if you need more inspiration to execute the progressions fundament you basically will fail.

Genetics

How significant your hereditary make-up is in arriving at your objective relies upon what objective you have set yourself and how your hereditary make-up finds a place with it.

The main comment is paying little mind to your hereditary history everyone is fit for building a body to be glad for with the correct preparing techniques, diet, and inspiration. The lone variable is that it can take more time for some than for other people.

Nonetheless, on the off chance that you need to be the new Arnold Schwarzenegger or Doreen Yates, I am apprehensive it is just the individuals who are adequately lucky to have the ideal hereditary qualities for building muscle that can make that degree of progress. While the facts confirm that these legends have extraordinary inspiration, drive and knowledge so do numerous other people who won't ever be as effective. Building muscle is simple however to be the best you need the best hereditary qualities. For instance, the incomplete tour De France rider Lance Armstrong's heart is 33%

greater than normal people. You can see he had the ideal hereditary qualities for his game.

Steroids

In my years as a gym center proprietor and educator, I have seen numerous youngsters put on a gigantic measure of muscle rapidly using steroids. Individuals who do go down this street won't ever acquire similar regard given to the individuals who have worked their bodies through difficult work and commitment and neither, should they?

Anything which can significantly adjust your body should likewise have emotional results. As the colloquialism goes, each activity has a response. If you question this look at the constant sickness and unexpected passing paces of the jocks of the 60s and 70s. Steroids are an unequivocal no, no.

Remember

You can assemble muscle with bodyweight practices on the off chance that you follow the standards of weight preparing and incorporate a similar number of activities, sets, redundancies, and constantly progress to additional requesting works out.

All muscle-building programs rely upon the right eating to guarantee achievement. If you have the devotion and inspiration to follow every one of these suggestions you will succeed and that is a logical reality. The lone variable is the time it will take the person.